ACID REFLUX COOKBOOK FOR BEGINNERS

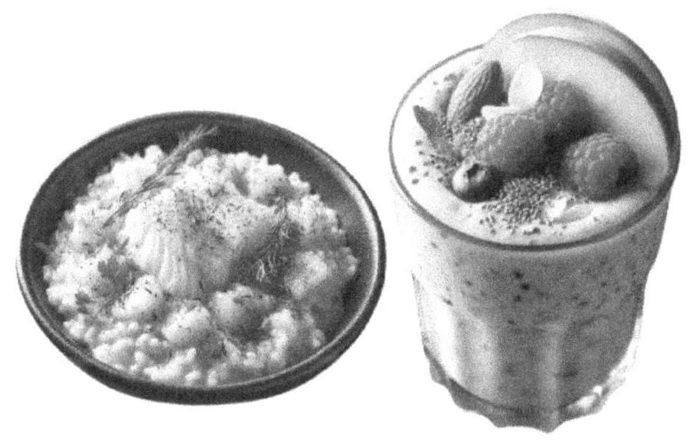

Easy and Delicious Recipes to Combat Acid Reflux

Lanita Cruz

TABLE OF CONTENT

DISCLAIMER

The information provided in this book is intended for general informational purposes only and should not be considered a substitute for professional medical advice. While we have taken great care to provide accurate and up-to-date information, it is essential to consult with a qualified healthcare professional before making significant dietary changes, especially if you have been diagnosed with any other medical condition.

The recipes in this cookbook have been designed to follow the principles of a Acid Reflux diet, but individual dietary requirements may vary. We encourage you to consider your health, preferences, and any food allergies or sensitivities when using these recipes.

The authors, publisher and any related parties do not assume responsibility for any adverse effects, allergic reactions, or health issues that may result from using or misusing the recipes or information provided in this cookbook.

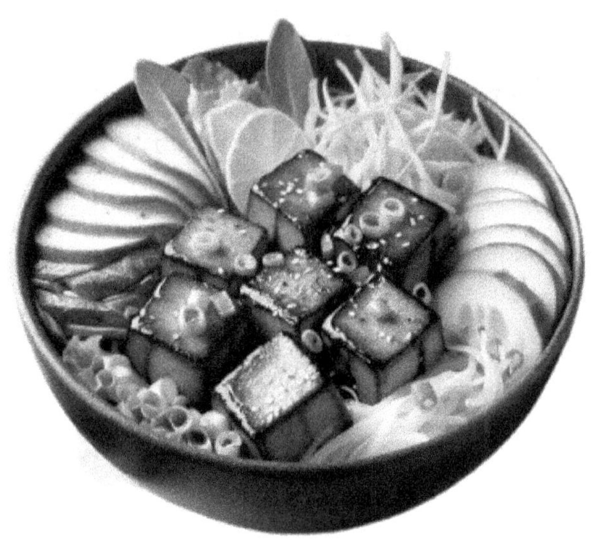

Introduction

If you've been grappling with the discomfort of acid reflux, you're not alone.

Acid reflux is a common condition that affects millions of people worldwide, it occurs when the stomach acid flows back into the esophagus, causing a burning sensation in the chest or throat.

This can lead to symptoms such as heartburn, regurgitation, nausea, bloating, and difficulty swallowing. If left untreated, acid reflux can damage the lining of the esophagus and increase the risk of esophageal cancer.

The good news is that acid reflux can be managed with dietary and lifestyle changes.

By avoiding foods that trigger or worsen the symptoms, and eating foods that soothe and heal the esophagus, you can reduce the frequency and severity of acid reflux episodes.

You can also improve your digestion and overall health by following some simple principles, such as eating smaller and more frequent meals, chewing your food well, drinking enough water, and avoiding smoking and alcohol.

In this book, you will find everything you need to know about the acid reflux diet, including the benefits, the foods to eat and avoid, and a comprehensive shopping list.

You will also discover delicious and easy recipes for breakfast, lunch, dinner, desserts, snacks, and beverages that are suitable for the acid reflux diet.

These recipes are designed to provide you with balanced nutrition, variety, and flavor, while keeping your acid reflux under control.

You will also get a 30-day meal plan that will help you plan your meals and stick to the diet.

Whether you have been diagnosed with acid reflux, or you just want to prevent it from happening, this book is for you.

It will help you enjoy your food without suffering from the consequences. With the acid reflux diet, you can say goodbye to heartburn and hello to a healthier and happier life.

CHAPTER 1

Principles of the Acid Reflux Diet

1. **Mindful Eating**: The acid reflux diet emphasizes the importance of mindful eating. Slow down, savor each bite, and pay attention to your body's signals, avoid overeating, as excess food can contribute to increased stomach pressure, triggering reflux.

2. **Balancing pH Levels**: Maintaining a balanced pH level in the stomach is a key principle. Include alkaline-rich foods, such as fruits and vegetables, to counteract acidic content. Striking this balance can help prevent the backflow of stomach acid into the esophagus.

3. **Portion Control:** Controlling portion sizes is vital to prevent excessive pressure on the lower esophageal sphincter (LES). Smaller, more frequent meals reduce the likelihood of stomach contents pushing upward, minimizing the risk of reflux.

4. **Identifying Trigger Foods:** Recognizing and avoiding trigger foods is paramount. Certain items, like spicy foods, citrus, and caffeine, can exacerbate

acid reflux. This section provides insights into common trigger foods, empowering you to make informed choices.

5. **Healthy Fats and Fiber:** Introducing healthy fats and fiber into the diet is encouraged. These elements aid in digestion and help maintain a healthy weight, reducing the likelihood of reflux. Avocados, nuts, and whole grains are examples of foods rich in these beneficial components.

6. **Hydration Habits:** Proper hydration is essential for digestive health. However, the timing of fluid intake matters. Consuming liquids between meals, rather than with them, helps prevent the dilution of stomach acid and minimizes the risk of reflux.

By embracing these principles, you can lay a solid groundwork for your acid reflux diet journey. Understanding how lifestyle and dietary choices impact digestive health is the first step towards finding relief and enjoying a more comfortable life.

Benefits of Acid Reflux Diet

1. **Reduced Symptoms**: The primary benefit of adopting an acid reflux diet is a significant reduction in symptoms. By avoiding trigger foods and following recommended dietary practices, you may experience less frequent and less severe episodes of heartburn, regurgitation, and other discomforts associated with acid reflux.

2. **Improved Digestive Health**: It encourages the consumption of nutrient-dense and easily digestible foods. This promotes overall digestive health by reducing the strain on the digestive system, leading to better nutrient absorption and improved gut function.

3. **Weight Management**: Following the principles of the acid reflux diet often leads to healthier eating habits and portion control. This, in turn, can contribute to weight management. Maintaining a healthy weight is crucial for preventing excessive pressure on the stomach and minimizing the risk of reflux.

4. **Enhanced Sleep Quality**: Acid reflux symptoms can disrupt sleep patterns, leading to discomfort and sleep disturbances. By making dietary adjustments and avoiding certain foods close to bedtime, you may experience improved sleep quality and fewer nighttime reflux episodes.

5. **Prevention of Complications**: Untreated or poorly managed acid reflux can lead to more severe complications such as esophagitis or Barrett's esophagus. Adhering to an acid reflux diet helps prevent these complications by addressing the root causes and reducing the likelihood of prolonged exposure to stomach acid.

6. **Increased Energy Levels**: A well-balanced acid reflux diet, rich in essential nutrients, can contribute to increased energy levels. Nutrient-dense foods provide the body with the fuel it needs for optimal functioning, helping you feel more energized and vibrant.

7. **Enhanced Quality of Life**: Ultimately, the acid reflux diet offers an improved quality of life. By understanding the positive impact of dietary choices

on symptoms and overall well-being, you can take control of your health and enjoy a more comfortable and fulfilling lifestyle.

Foods to Eat

Lean Proteins: Opt for lean sources of protein such as chicken, turkey, fish & tofu. These protein-rich choices minimize the risk of stomach acid overproduction, promoting better digestion.

Vegetables: Incorporate a variety of colorful vegetables into your diet, focusing on non-acidic options like leafy greens, broccoli, carrots & cauliflower. These vegetables provide essential nutrients without exacerbating acid reflux.

Whole Grains: Choose whole grains over refined grains for a fiber boost. Oats, brown rice, quinoa, and whole-grain bread are excellent choices, aiding in digestion and helping maintain a healthy weight.

Non-Citrus Fruits: Opt for non-citrus fruits such as bananas, melons, apples, and pears. These fruits offer natural sweetness and essential vitamins without contributing to acid reflux symptoms.

Healthy Fats: Incorporate sources of healthy fats, including nuts, avocados & olive oil. These fats support overall health and can be included in moderation to add flavor and richness to your meals.

Dairy Alternatives: If dairy triggers your acid reflux, explore non-dairy alternatives like almond milk or oat milk. These options provide a creamy texture without the acidity found in traditional dairy products.

Herbs and Spices: Flavor your dishes with herbs and mild spices such as basil, parsley, ginger, and turmeric. These additions not only enhance taste but also offer potential anti-inflammatory benefits.

Low-Acid Beverages: Stay hydrated with water, herbal teas, and non-citrus infused water. Hydration is crucial for digestive health, and these options help maintain the delicate balance in the stomach.

Foods to Avoid

Citrus Fruits: Citrus fruits like oranges, grapefruits, and lemons are highly acidic and can stimulate acid production.

Avoiding these fruits can help reduce the risk of acid reflux episodes.

Tomatoes and Tomato-Based Products: Tomatoes are naturally acidic, and their acidity can contribute to heartburn. Steer clear of tomato-based sauces, ketchup, and marinades to minimize the impact on acid reflux symptoms.

Spicy Foods: Spices, particularly those with heat such as chili and black pepper, can irritate the esophagus and trigger acid reflux. Opt for milder herbs and spices to season your dishes.

High-Fat Foods: Fatty foods, including fried items, full-fat dairy, and rich sauces, can relax the lower esophageal sphincter (LES) and promote the flow of stomach acid into the esophagus. Opt for leaner alternatives to minimize this risk.

Chocolate: While delicious, chocolate contains substances that can relax the LES, making it easier for stomach acid to flow back into the esophagus. Consider indulging in moderation or exploring carob as a chocolate substitute.

Mint and Peppermint: While often associated with digestive relief, mint and peppermint can relax the LES and contribute to acid reflux. Choose alternative flavors for teas and avoid excessive consumption of mint-flavored products.

Onions and Garlic: Onions and garlic are known to cause digestive discomfort, and they can worsen acid reflux symptoms. Experiment with milder herbs and flavorings to add depth to your dishes.

Caffeine and Carbonated Beverages: Coffee, tea, and carbonated drinks can contribute to acid reflux by relaxing the LES and increasing stomach acid production. Opt for herbal teas and non-acidic, non-caffeinated alternatives.

Comprehensive Shopping List for Acid Reflux Diet

Proteins:

- Skinless poultry (chicken, turkey)
- Fish (salmon, trout, cod)
- Tofu

- Lean cuts of beef or pork (in moderation)

Vegetables:

- Leafy greens (spinach, kale, Swiss chard)
- Broccoli
- Cauliflower
- Carrots
- Zucchini
- Sweet potatoes

Whole Grains:

- Oats
- Brown rice
- Quinoa
- Whole-grain bread
- Barley

Non-Citrus Fruits:

- Bananas
- Melons (watermelon, cantaloupe)
- Apples
- Pears

Healthy Fats:

- Avocados
- Nuts (almonds, walnuts)
- Olive oil

Dairy Alternatives:

- Almond milk
- Oat milk

Herbs and Spices:

- Basil
- Parsley
- Ginger
- Turmeric
- Cumin

CHAPTER 2

Breakfast Recipes for Acid Reflux Diet

Tropical Oatmeal

- **Preparation Time:** 10 minutes
- **Serves:** 2

Ingredients:

- 1 cup rolled oats
- 1 ½ cups coconut milk
- 1 ripe banana, sliced
- ½ cup fresh pineapple chunks
- 1 tablespoon chia seeds
- 1 tablespoon shredded coconut
- 1 tablespoon honey

Nutritional Information: Calories: 380 | Protein: 7g | Fat: 15g | Carbohydrates: 56g | Fiber: 9g

Instructions:

1. In a saucepan, combine rolled oats and coconut milk.

2. Cook over medium heat, stirring occasionally, until oats reach desired consistency.

3. Once cooked, divide the oatmeal into two bowls.

4. Top with sliced banana, fresh pineapple chunks, chia seeds, shredded coconut, and a drizzle of honey.

5. Gently mix the toppings into the oatmeal.

6. Serve warm.

Serving Suggestions:

- Garnish with a sprinkle of extra shredded coconut for added texture.

- Pair with a refreshing glass of coconut water or herbal tea for a complete tropical breakfast experience.

Whole Grain English Muffin

- **Preparation Time:** 15 minutes
- **Serves:** 2

Ingredients:

- 2 whole grain English muffins, split and toasted

- 2 poached eggs

- 1 avocado, sliced

- 1 tablespoon olive oil

- Salt and pepper to taste

- Optional: Fresh herbs for garnish

Nutritional Information: Calories: 320 | Protein: 12g | Fat: 18g | Carbohydrates: 28g | Fiber: 8g

Instructions:

1. Toast the whole grain English muffins to your liking.
2. In a skillet, heat olive oil over medium heat, poach the eggs until whites are set but yolks remain runny.
3. Place a poached egg on each toasted muffin half.
4. Top with sliced avocado, salt, and pepper.
5. Garnish with fresh herbs if desired.
6. Serve immediately.

Serving Suggestions:

- Sprinkle a dash of hot sauce for extra flavor.

- Serve alongside a side of mixed berries for a balanced and satisfying meal.

Fabulous French Toast

- **Preparation Time:** 20 minutes
- **Serves:** 4

Ingredients:

- 8 slices whole grain bread
- 2 large eggs
- 1 cup almond milk
- 1 teaspoon vanilla extract
- 1 teaspoon ground cinnamon
- 1 tablespoon coconut oil
- Fresh berries for topping

Nutritional Information: Calories: 220 | Protein: 9g | Fat: 8g | Carbohydrates: 30g | Fiber: 6g

Instructions:

- Whisk eggs, vanilla extract, almond milk, and ground cinnamon together in a bowl.
- Heat coconut oil in a skillet over medium heat, dip each slice of bread into the egg mixture, coating both sides.

- Cook the slices until golden brown on each side.

- Arrange French toast on plates and top with fresh berries.

- Optional: Drizzle with a touch of honey for sweetness.

Serving Suggestions:

- Dust with a sprinkle of powdered sugar for a delightful finish.

- Serve with a side of Greek yogurt for added protein.

Easy Vegan Quinoa Breakfast

- **Preparation Time:** 15 minutes
- **Serves:** 2

Ingredients:

- 1 cup cooked quinoa
- 1 cup almond milk
- 1 tablespoon maple syrup
- 1/2 teaspoon ground cinnamon
- 1/2 cup mixed berries
- 2 tablespoons chopped nuts (almonds, walnuts)

- Fresh mint leaves for garnish

Nutritional Information: Calories: 280 | Protein: 7g | Fat: 8g | Carbohydrates: 45g | Fiber: 6g

Instructions:

1. In a saucepan, warm the cooked quinoa with almond milk over medium heat.
2. Stir in maple syrup and ground cinnamon.
3. Once heated through, divide the quinoa mixture into bowls.
4. Top with mixed berries and chopped nuts.
5. Garnish with fresh mint leaves.
6. Serve warm.

Serving Suggestions:

- Add a dollop of coconut yogurt for creaminess.
- Sprinkle a pinch of chia seeds for an extra nutritional boost.

Skillet Harvest Pumpkin Hash

- **Preparation Time:** 25 minutes
- **Serves:** 3

Ingredients:

- 2 cups diced pumpkin
- 1 sweet potato, peeled and diced
- 1 red bell pepper, diced
- 1 small red onion, finely chopped
- 2 tablespoons olive oil
- 1 teaspoon smoked paprika
- 1/2 teaspoon ground cumin
- Salt and pepper to taste
- 3 poached eggs (optional)

Nutritional Information: Calories: 180 | Protein: 3g | Fat: 8g | Carbohydrates: 25g | Fiber: 5g

Instructions:

1. In a skillet, heat olive oil over medium heat, add diced pumpkin, sweet potato, red bell pepper, and red onion to the skillet.
2. Sprinkle with smoked paprika, ground cumin, salt, and pepper.
3. Cook, stirring occasionally, until vegetables are tender.

4. If desired, poach eggs in a separate pan.

5. Serve the pumpkin hash with or without poached eggs on top.

Serving Suggestions:

- Decorate with fresh herbs like parsley or cilantro.

- You can serve with a side of sliced avocado for added creaminess.

Grain Free Cinnamon Apple Granola

- **Preparation Time:** 30 minutes
- **Serves:** 4

Ingredients:

- 2 cups mixed nuts (almonds, walnuts, pecans), chopped

- 1 cup unsweetened coconut flakes

- 1 cup dried apple slices, chopped

- 2 tablespoons coconut oil, melted

- 1 tablespoon maple syrup

- 1 teaspoon ground cinnamon

- 1/2 teaspoon vanilla extract

- A pinch of salt

Nutritional Information: Calories: 280 | Protein: 7g | Fat: 24g | Carbohydrates: 12g | Fiber: 5g

Instructions:

1. Preheat the oven to 300°F (150°C) and line a baking sheet with parchment paper.
2. In a large bowl, combine chopped nuts, coconut flakes, and dried apple slices.
3. In a separate bowl, mix melted coconut oil, maple syrup, ground cinnamon, vanilla extract, and a pinch of salt.
4. Pour the wet mixture over the dry ingredients and toss until evenly coated.
5. Spread the mixture onto the prepared baking sheet in an even layer.
6. Bake for 20-25 minutes, stirring halfway through, or until golden brown and fragrant.
7. Allow the granola to cool completely before storing in an airtight container.

Serving Suggestions:

- Enjoy with your favorite non-dairy yogurt.
- Sprinkle over a bowl of fresh berries for a nutritious breakfast.

Maple Sage Breakfast Patties

- **Preparation Time:** 20 minutes
- **Serves:** 3

Ingredients:

- 1 lb lean ground turkey
- 1/4 cup of fresh sage leaves, finely chopped
- 2 tablespoons pure maple syrup
- 1 teaspoon ground black pepper
- 1/2 teaspoon salt
- 1/2 teaspoon garlic powder
- 1/4 teaspoon smoked paprika
- 1 tablespoon olive oil (for cooking)

Nutritional Information: Calories: 210 | Protein: 25g | Fat: 10g | Carbohydrates: 5g | Fiber: 1g

Instructions:

1. In a mixing bowl, combine ground turkey, chopped sage, maple syrup, black pepper, salt, garlic powder, and smoked paprika.
2. Mix the ingredients thoroughly until it is well combined.
3. Divide the mixture into small portions and shape them into patties.
4. Heat olive oil in a skillet over medium heat, cook the patties for 4-5 minutes on each side or until fully cooked and browned.
5. Ensure the internal temperature reaches 165°F (74°C).
6. Remove from the skillet and let them rest for a couple of minutes before serving.

Serving Suggestions:

- Serve with a side of sautéed spinach or a mixed green salad.
- Enjoy with a dollop of plain Greek yogurt for added creaminess.

Lunch Recipes for Acid Reflux Diet

Tortilla Wrap with Baked Omelet

- **Preparation Time:** 15 minutes
- **Serves:** 2

Ingredients:

- 4 large eggs
- 1/4 cup milk
- Salt and pepper to taste
- 1 cup baby spinach, chopped
- 1/2 cup cherry tomatoes, halved
- 1/4 cup feta cheese, crumbled
- 2 whole-grain tortillas
- Cooking spray

Nutritional Information: Calories: 350 | Protein: 20g | Fat: 18g | Carbohydrates: 28g | Fiber: 5g

Instructions:

1. Preheat the oven to 375°F (190°C).
2. In a bowl, whisk together eggs, milk, salt, and pepper.

3. Stir in chopped spinach, halved cherry tomatoes, and crumbled feta cheese.

4. Spray an oven-safe skillet with cooking spray and pour the egg mixture into it.

5. Bake in the preheated oven for 10-12 minutes or until the omelet is set.

6. Remove the skillet from the oven and let the omelet cool slightly.

7. Place a tortilla on a flat surface and add half of the baked omelet.

8. Roll the tortilla, enclosing the omelet.

9. Repeat the process for the second tortilla.

10. Optionally, slice each wrap in half for easier handling.

Serving Suggestions:

- Serve with a side of fresh salsa or Greek yogurt.
- Pair with a mixed green salad for a complete and satisfying lunch.

Couscous with Cod Fish

- **Preparation Time:** 20 minutes
- **Serves:** 2

Ingredients:

- 1 cup whole wheat couscous
- 1 cup cherry tomatoes, halved
- 1/2 cup cucumber, diced
- 1/4 cup red onion, finely chopped
- 2 cod fish fillets
- 2 tablespoons olive oil
- 1 lemon, juiced
- 1 teaspoon dried oregano
- Salt and pepper to taste
- Fresh parsley for garnish

Nutritional Information: Calories: 420 | Protein: 30g | Fat: 15g | Carbohydrates: 40g | Fiber: 6g

Instructions:

1. Cook couscous according to package instructions.

2. In a bowl, combine halved cherry tomatoes, diced cucumber, and finely chopped red onion.

3. Season the cod fish fillets with olive oil, lemon juice, dried oregano, salt, and pepper.

4. Grill or bake the cod fillets until fully cooked.

5. Fluff the cooked couscous with a fork and divide it onto plates.

6. Top with the vegetable mixture and place a grilled cod fillet on each plate.

7. Garnish with fresh parsley.

Serving Suggestions:

- Drizzle with extra lemon juice for a citrusy kick.
- You can serve with a side of steamed broccoli or a green salad.

Lunch Burger

- **Preparation Time:** 25 minutes
- **Serves:** 2

Ingredients:

- 1/2 lb lean ground turkey

- 1 tablespoon olive oil
- 1/2 teaspoon garlic powder
- Salt and pepper to taste
- 2 whole grain burger buns
- 1 avocado, sliced
- Lettuce leaves
- Tomato slices
- Red onion rings

Nutritional Information: Calories: 380 | Protein: 25g | Fat: 15g | Carbohydrates: 35g | Fiber: 8g

Instructions:

1. In a bowl, mix ground turkey with garlic powder, salt, and pepper.
2. Form the turkey mixture into two burger patties.
3. Heat olive oil in a skillet over medium heat, cook the burger patties for 5-6 minutes on each side or until fully cooked.
4. Toast the whole grain burger buns.
5. Assemble the burgers with sliced avocado, lettuce, tomato, and red onion.

Serving Suggestions:

- Serve with a side of oven-baked sweet potato wedges.
- You can add a dollop of Greek yogurt or tzatziki sauce for extra creaminess.

Sweet White Rice Pudding

- **Preparation Time:** 30 minutes
- **Serves:** 4

Ingredients:

- 1 cup Arborio rice
- 4 cups almond milk
- 1/3 cup honey or maple syrup
- 1 teaspoon vanilla extract
- 1/2 teaspoon ground cinnamon
- 1/4 cup raisins (optional)
- Sliced almonds for garnish

Nutritional Information: Calories: 250 | Protein: 4g | Fat: 2g | Carbohydrates: 55g | Fiber: 2g

Instructions:

1. Rinse Arborio rice under cold water.

2. In a saucepan, combine rice, almond milk, honey or maple syrup, vanilla extract, and ground cinnamon.

3. Bring to a gentle simmer over medium heat, stirring occasionally.

4. Cook for 20-25 minutes or until the rice is tender and the mixture has thickened.

5. Stir in raisins if desired and cook for an additional 5 minutes.

6. Remove from heat and let it cool slightly before serving, garnish with sliced almonds.

Serving Suggestions:

- Sprinkle a dash of ground cinnamon on top.
- Serve warm or chilled, depending on your preference.

Bacon, Pear, and Fig Grilled Cheese

- **Preparation Time:** 15 minutes
- **Serves:** 2

Ingredients:

- 4 slices whole grain bread
- 4 slices bacon, cooked
- 1 ripe pear, thinly sliced
- 4 dried figs, sliced
- 1 cup shredded sharp cheddar cheese
- Butter for spreading

Nutritional Information: Calories: 480 | Protein: 20g | Fat: 25g | Carbohydrates: 45g | Fiber: 8g

Instructions:

1. Lay out the slices of bread.
2. On two slices, evenly distribute the cooked bacon, pear slices, dried figs, and shredded cheddar.
3. Top with the remaining slices of bread to create sandwiches.
4. Spread butter on the outer sides of each sandwich.
5. Heat a skillet over medium heat, grill the sandwiches until the bread is golden brown, and the cheese is melted.
6. Slice the sandwiches in half diagonally.

Serving Suggestions:

- Serve with a side of mixed greens dressed with balsamic vinaigrette.
- Pair with a warm cup of herbal tea or a light soup.

White Bean & Avocado Toast

- **Preparation Time:** 10 minutes
- **Serves:** 2

Ingredients:

- 15 oz (1 can) white beans, rinsed & drained
- 1 clove garlic, minced
- 2 tablespoons lemon juice
- Salt and pepper to taste
- 4 slices whole grain bread, toasted
- 1 ripe avocado, sliced
- Red pepper flakes for garnish (optional)
- Fresh cilantro for garnish (optional)

Nutritional Information: Calories: 320 | Protein: 12g | Fat: 14g | Carbohydrates: 40g | Fiber: 12g

Instructions:

1. In a bowl, mash white beans with minced garlic, lemon juice, salt, and pepper.
2. Toast the whole grain bread slices.
3. Spread the mashed white beans evenly over the toasted bread.
4. Top with sliced avocado.
5. Garnish with red pepper flakes and fresh cilantro if desired.
6. Serve immediately.

Serving Suggestions:

- You can drizzle with a touch of extra virgin olive oil.
- Sprinkle with a pinch of sea salt for enhanced flavor.

Rainbow Veggie Wraps

- **Preparation Time:** 20 minutes
- **Serves:** 2

Ingredients:

- 4 whole grain tortillas

- Hummus for spreading

- 1 cup shredded red cabbage

- 1 bell pepper, thinly sliced (assorted colors)

- 1 large carrot, julienned

- 1 zucchini, sliced into thin strips

- 1/2 cup cherry tomatoes, halved

- 1/4 cup fresh cilantro, chopped

- 1 tablespoon olive oil

- Salt and pepper to taste

Nutritional Information: Calories: 300 | Protein: 8g | Fat: 10g | Carbohydrates: 45g | Fiber: 8g

Instructions:

1. Lay out the whole grain tortillas on a flat surface.

2. Spread a generous layer of hummus on each tortilla.

3. Evenly distribute shredded red cabbage, bell pepper slices, julienned carrot, zucchini strips, cherry tomato halves, and chopped cilantro among the tortillas.

4. Drizzle olive oil over the veggies and sprinkle with salt and pepper.

5. Roll the tortillas tightly to create wraps.

6. Slice the wraps in half diagonally.

Serving Suggestions:

- You can serve with a side of Greek yogurt or tzatziki sauce.

- Pair with a refreshing cucumber and mint-infused water.

Dinner Recipes for Acid Reflux Diet

Vegetarian Sausage with Braised Cabbage

- **Preparation Time:** 30 minutes
- **Serves:** 4

Ingredients:

- 8 vegetarian sausages

- 1 head green cabbage, shredded

- 1 onion, thinly sliced

- 2 apples, cored and sliced

- 2 tablespoons olive oil

- 1/4 cup apple cider vinegar

- 1 tablespoon Dijon mustard

- Salt and pepper to taste

- Fresh parsley for garnish

Nutritional Information: Calories: 350 | Protein: 15g | Fat: 20g | Carbohydrates: 30g | Fiber: 8g

Instructions:

1. In a large skillet, heat olive oil over medium heat, add vegetarian sausages and cook until browned on all sides.
2. Remove sausages from the skillet and set aside.
3. In the same skillet, add sliced onions and cook until softened.
4. Add shredded cabbage and sliced apples to the skillet, stirring to combine.
5. Pour in apple cider vinegar and Dijon mustard, mixing well.
6. Season with salt and pepper to your preferred taste.
7. Place the cooked sausages on top of the cabbage mixture.

8. Cover the skillet and let it simmer for 15-20 minutes or until the cabbage is tender.

9. Garnish with fresh parsley before serving.

Serving Suggestions:

- Serve over a bed of mashed sweet potatoes or cauliflower.

- Pair with a side of whole-grain mustard for extra flavor.

Polenta with Sesame Seeds

- **Preparation Time:** 25 minutes
- **Serves:** 4

Ingredients:

- 1 cup polenta
- 4 cups vegetable broth
- 2 tablespoons sesame seeds
- 2 tablespoons olive oil
- Salt and pepper to taste
- Chopped fresh chives for garnish

Nutritional Information: Calories: 280 | Protein: 5g | Fat: 10g | Carbohydrates: 40g | Fiber: 3g

Instructions:

1. In a saucepan, bring vegetable broth to a boil, gradually whisk in polenta, stirring continuously to avoid lumps.
2. Reduce heat to low and simmer, stirring occasionally, until the polenta is creamy.
3. Toast sesame seeds in a dry skillet over medium heat until golden brown.
4. Stir toasted sesame seeds into the polenta.
5. Drizzle with olive oil and season with salt and pepper to your preferred state.
6. Continue to stir until well combined.
7. Serve the polenta in bowls, garnished with chopped fresh chives.

Serving Suggestions:

- Top with sautéed mushrooms for an earthy flavor.

- Pair with a side of roasted vegetables for a complete meal.

Apricot Glazed Chicken

- **Preparation Time:** 35 minutes
- **Serves:** 4

Ingredients:

- 4 boneless, skinless chicken breasts
- Salt and pepper to taste
- 1 tablespoon olive oil
- 1/2 cup apricot preserves
- 2 tablespoons Dijon mustard
- 1 tablespoon soy sauce
- 2 cloves garlic, minced
- 1 teaspoon fresh ginger, grated
- Chopped fresh parsley for garnish

Nutritional Information: Calories: 320 | Protein: 30g | Fat: 8g | Carbohydrates: 25g | Fiber: 1g

Instructions:

1.   Season your chicken breasts with salt & pepper.

2.   In a large skillet, heat olive oil over medium-high heat, add chicken breasts and cook until browned on both sides and cooked through.

3.   In a small bowl, mix apricot preserves, Dijon mustard, soy sauce, minced garlic, and grated ginger.

4.   Pour the apricot glaze over the cooked chicken.

5.   Allow the glaze to simmer and coat the chicken for 3-4 minutes.

6.   Decorate with chopped fresh parsley before serving.

Serving Suggestions:

- Serve over a bed of quinoa or brown rice.
- Pair with steamed broccoli or green beans for a balanced meal.

Banh Mi Bowls with Sticky Tofu

- **Preparation Time:** 40 minutes
- **Serves:** 4

Ingredients:

- 1 cup jasmine rice, cooked
- 1 block extra-firm tofu, pressed and cubed
- 1/4 cup soy sauce
- 2 tablespoons hoisin sauce
- 1 tablespoon maple syrup
- 2 teaspoons sesame oil
- 1 cucumber, thinly sliced
- 2 carrots, julienned
- 1 cup radishes, thinly sliced
- Fresh cilantro for garnish
- Sriracha for serving (optional)

Nutritional Information: Calories: 380 | Protein: 15g | Fat: 10g | Carbohydrates: 60g | Fiber: 5g

Instructions:

1. In a bowl, mix soy sauce, hoisin sauce, maple syrup, and sesame oil.
2. Toss cubed tofu in the sauce mixture and let it marinate for 15 minutes.
3. Cook marinated tofu in a skillet over medium-high heat until sticky and golden brown.

4. Assemble bowls with cooked jasmine rice, sticky tofu, cucumber slices, julienned carrots, and sliced radishes.

5. Garnish with fresh cilantro.

6. Serve with sriracha on the side if you like it spicy.

Serving Suggestions:

- Drizzle with additional hoisin sauce for extra flavor.

Green Pizza with Pesto, Feta, Artichokes & Broccoli

- **Preparation Time:** 30 minutes
- **Serves:** 4

Ingredients:

- 1 pound whole wheat pizza dough
- 1/2 cup pesto sauce
- 1 cup broccoli florets, blanched
- 1/2 cup marinated artichoke hearts, drained and sliced
- 1/2 cup crumbled feta cheese
- 1/4 cup pine nuts

- Fresh basil for garnish

Nutritional Information: Calories: 420 | Protein: 15g | Fat: 15g | Carbohydrates: 55g | Fiber: 8g

Instructions:

1. Preheat the oven according to pizza dough instructions.
2. Roll out the pizza dough on a floured surface, spread pesto sauce evenly over the pizza dough.
3. Arrange blanched broccoli, sliced artichoke hearts, and crumbled feta on top.
4. Sprinkle pine nuts over the pizza.
5. Bake in the preheated oven until the crust is golden and toppings are bubbly.
6. Garnish with fresh basil before serving.

Serving Suggestions:

- Drizzle with a balsamic glaze for added sweetness.
- Serve with a side of mixed greens dressed with lemon vinaigrette.

Seared Scallops with Acorn Squash Mash

- **Preparation Time:** 25 minutes
- **Serves:** 4

Ingredients:

- 16 large sea scallops
- Salt and pepper to taste
- 2 tablespoons olive oil
- 2 acorn squashes, peeled, seeded, and diced
- 1/4 cup unsweetened almond milk
- 1 tablespoon fresh thyme leaves
- 1 tablespoon lemon zest
- Chopped fresh parsley for garnish

Nutritional Information: Calories: 280 | Protein: 20g | Fat: 12g | Carbohydrates: 25g | Fiber: 6g

Instructions:

1. Pat scallops dry and season with salt and pepper.

2. Heat olive oil in a skillet over medium-high heat, sear scallops for 2-3 minutes on each side or until golden brown and cooked through.

3. In a separate pot, steam diced acorn squash until tender.

4. Mash the steamed squash and mix in almond milk, fresh thyme, and lemon zest.

5. Season the squash mash with salt and pepper to taste.

6. Serve the seared scallops on a bed of acorn squash mash.

7. Garnish with chopped fresh parsley.

Serving Suggestions:

- Pair with a side of sautéed spinach or kale.
- Drizzle with a lemon-butter sauce for extra richness.

Mediterranean Farro Salad with Arugula and Chickpeas

- **Preparation Time:** 30 minutes
- **Serves:** 4

Ingredients:

- 1 cup farro, cooked and cooled
- 2 cups arugula
- 15 oz (1 can) of chickpeas, rinsed and drained
- 1 cup cherry tomatoes, halved
- 1/2 cup Kalamata olives, sliced
- 1/4 cup red onion, finely chopped
- 1/2 cup feta cheese, crumbled
- 2 tablespoons extra virgin olive oil
- 1 tablespoon balsamic vinegar
- Salt and pepper to taste

Nutritional Information: Calories: 320 | Protein: 12g | Fat: 15g | Carbohydrates: 40g | Fiber: 8g

Instructions:

1. In a large bowl, combine cooked farro, arugula, chickpeas, cherry tomatoes, Kalamata olives, red onion, and feta cheese.
2. In a small bowl, whisk together extra virgin olive oil and balsamic vinegar.

3. Pour the dressing over the salad and toss until well coated.

4. Season with salt and pepper to your preferred taste.

5. Serve the Mediterranean farro salad chilled.

Serving Suggestions:

- You can top with grilled chicken or shrimp for added protein.

- Serve with a side of whole-grain pita bread or a light soup.

Desserts and Snacks for Acid Reflux Diet

Coconut & Cacao Loaf

- **Preparation Time:** 15 minutes
- **Serves:** 8

Ingredients:

- 1 1/2 cups almond flour
- 1/2 cup coconut flour
- 1/2 cup cacao powder

- 1 teaspoon baking soda

- 1/4 teaspoon salt

- 3 large eggs

- 1/2 cup coconut oil, melted

- 1/2 cup maple syrup

- 1 teaspoon vanilla extract

- 1 cup unsweetened almond milk

- 1/2 cup shredded coconut (unsweetened)

Nutritional Information: Calories: 280 | Protein: 8g | Fat: 20g | Carbohydrates: 20g | Fiber: 6g

Instructions:

1. Preheat the oven to 350°F (175°C), grease a loaf pan.

2. In a large bowl, whisk together almond flour, coconut flour, cacao powder, baking soda, and salt.

3. In a separate bowl, beat the eggs and add melted coconut oil, maple syrup, and vanilla extract. Mix well.

4. Gradually add the wet ingredients to the dry ingredients, stirring until combined.

5. Pour in almond milk and continue to mix until a smooth batter forms.

6. Fold in shredded coconut.

7. Transfer the batter to the greased loaf pan and smooth the top.

8. Bake for 42-45 minutes or until the toothpick inserted into the center comes out clean.

9. Allow the loaf to cool in the pan for 10 minutes before transferring it to a wire rack to cool completely.

Serving Suggestions:

- You can slice and serve with a dollop of coconut yogurt.
- Garnish with fresh berries for a burst of color and flavor.

Paleo Vanilla Sponge Cake

- **Preparation Time:** 20 minutes
- **Serves:** 8

Ingredients:

- 2 cups almond flour

- 1/4 cup coconut flour

- 1 teaspoon baking soda

- Pinch of salt

- 4 large eggs

- 1/2 cup coconut oil, melted

- 1/2 cup maple syrup

- 1 tablespoon vanilla extract

- Fresh berries for garnish

Nutritional Information: Calories: 240 | Protein: 8g | Fat: 18g | Carbohydrates: 15g | Fiber: 3g

Instructions:

1. Preheat the oven to 350°F (175°C) and grease your round cake pan.

2. In a large bowl, combine almond flour, coconut flour, baking soda, and a pinch of salt.

3. In a separate bowl, whisk together eggs, melted coconut oil, maple syrup, and vanilla extract.

4. Gradually add the wet ingredients to the dry one, continue stirring until smooth.

5. Pour the batter into the prepared cake pan and spread it evenly.

6. Bake for 25-30 minutes or until the toothpick you inserted into the center comes out clean.

7. Allow the cake to cool in the pan for 10 minutes before you transfer it to a wire rack to cool completely.

Serving Suggestions:

- Top with a dusting of coconut flour for a decorative touch.

- Serve with a side of whipped coconut cream and fresh berries.

Cherry & Almond Clafoutis

- **Preparation Time:** 15 minutes
- **Serves:** 6

Ingredients:

- 2 cups fresh cherries, pitted
- 1/2 cup almond flour
- 1/4 cup coconut flour

- 1/4 cup maple syrup

- 3 large eggs

- 1 cup almond milk

- 1 teaspoon almond extract

- Pinch of salt

- Sliced almonds for garnish

Nutritional Information: Calories: 180 | Protein: 6g | Fat: 10g | Carbohydrates: 20g | Fiber: 4g

Instructions:

1. Preheat the oven to 350°F (175°C) and grease your baking dish.

2. Arrange pitted cherries in a single layer in the baking dish.

3. In a bowl, whisk together almond flour, coconut flour, maple syrup, eggs, almond milk, almond extract, and a pinch of salt until well combined.

4. Pour the batter over the cherries in the baking dish, bake for 25-30 minutes or until the clafoutis is set and golden brown.

5. Allow it to cool slightly before serving, garnish with sliced almonds.

Serving Suggestions:

- Dust with a bit of powdered sugar for an extra touch.
- Serve warm with a scoop of dairy-free vanilla ice cream.

Blueberry Banana Smoothie

- **Preparation Time:** 5 minutes
- **Serves:** 2

Ingredients:

- 1 cup frozen blueberries
- 1 ripe banana
- 1 cup almond milk
- 1 tablespoon almond butter
- 1 teaspoon chia seeds
- Ice cubes (optional)

Nutritional Information: Calories: 180 | Protein: 4g | Fat: 8g | Carbohydrates: 25g | Fiber: 6g

Instructions:

1. In a blender, combine frozen blueberries, ripe banana, almond milk, almond butter, and chia seeds.
2. Blend until it is smooth and creamy.
3. Add ice cubes if a colder consistency is desired and blend again.
4. Pour into glasses and serve immediately.

Serving Suggestions:

- Garnish with a few whole blueberries for a burst of freshness.
- Sprinkle with additional chia seeds for added texture.

Bagel and Lox

- **Preparation Time:** 10 minutes
- **Serves:** 2

Ingredients:

- 2 gluten-free bagels
- 4 oz smoked salmon (lox)
- 1/2 cup dairy-free cream cheese
- 1 tablespoon capers
- 1/4 red onion, thinly sliced
- Fresh dill for garnish

Nutritional Information: Calories: 350 | Protein: 18g | Fat: 15g | Carbohydrates: 40g | Fiber: 5g

Instructions:

1. Slice the gluten-free bagels in half and toast them if desired.
2. Spread dairy-free cream cheese on each bagel half.
3. Arrange smoked salmon on top of the cream cheese.
4. Sprinkle capers and thinly sliced red onion over the salmon.
5. Garnish with fresh dill.
6. Serve immediately.

Serving Suggestions:

- Accompany with lemon wedges for a citrusy kick.
- Serve with a side of mixed greens for a well-rounded snack or light meal.

Beverages/Drinks for Acid Reflux Diet

Cinnamon Cashew Milk

- **Preparation Time:** 10 minutes
- **Serves:** 4

Ingredients:

- 1 cup raw cashews, soaked overnight
- 4 cups filtered water
- 2 tablespoons maple syrup
- 1 teaspoon ground cinnamon
- 1 teaspoon vanilla extract
- Pinch of salt

Nutritional Information: Calories: 120 | Protein: 3g | Fat: 8g | Carbohydrates: 10g | Fiber: 1g

Instructions:

1. Drain and rinse soaked cashews.

2. In a blender, combine cashews, filtered water, maple syrup, ground cinnamon, vanilla extract, and a pinch of salt.

3. Blend on high speed until smooth and well combined.

4. Strain the mixture through a nut milk bag or fine mesh sieve into a bowl, separating the liquid from the pulp.

5. Transfer the strained cashew milk to a bottle or container.

6. Refrigerate until chilled.

7. Shake well before serving.

Serving Suggestions:

- You can serve over ice for a refreshing drink.
- Use in coffee or tea as a dairy-free creamer.

Licorice Tea

- **Preparation Time:** 5 minutes
- **Serves:** 2

Ingredients:

- 2 licorice tea bags

- 2 cups boiling water

- 1 tablespoon honey (optional)

- Slices of fresh ginger (optional)

- Lemon slices for garnish

Nutritional Information: Calories: 5 | Protein: 0g | Fat: 0g | Carbohydrates: 1g | Fiber: 0g

Instructions:

1. Place licorice tea bags in a teapot or heatproof pitcher.
2. Pour boiling water over the tea bags.
3. Allow the tea to steep for 4-5 minutes.
4. Remove the tea bags and sweeten with honey if desired.
5. Add slices of fresh ginger for an extra kick (optional).
6. Pour into cups and garnish with lemon slices.

Serving Suggestions:

- Enjoy warm or over ice.

- Pair with a light, acid reflux-friendly snack

Apple Cider Vinegar Drink

- **Preparation Time:** 5 minutes
- **Serves:** 1

Ingredients:

- 1 tablespoon of apple cider vinegar (raw, unfiltered)
- 1 cup water
- 1 tablespoon honey
- 1/2 teaspoon grated fresh ginger
- Pinch of cayenne pepper (optional)

Nutritional Information: Calories: 30 | Protein: 0g | Fat: 0g | Carbohydrates: 8g | Fiber: 0g

Instructions:

1. In a glass, mix apple cider vinegar with water.
2. Add honey and stir until well dissolved.
3. Grate fresh ginger into the mixture and stir.
4. For a bit of heat, add a pinch of cayenne pepper (optional).
5. Stir well and drink immediately.

Serving Suggestions:

- Consume 15-20 minutes before meals to aid digestion.
- Adjust honey to taste for sweetness.

Mango Lassi

- **Preparation Time:** 10 minutes
- **Serves:** 2

Ingredients:

- 1 cup ripe mango (peeled & diced)
- 1 cup dairy-free yogurt
- 1/2 cup almond milk
- 2 tablespoons maple syrup
- 1/2 teaspoon ground cardamom
- Ice cubes (optional)

Nutritional Information: Calories: 180 | Protein: 4g | Fat: 8g | Carbohydrates: 25g | Fiber: 3g

Instructions:

1. In a blender, combine diced mango, dairy-free yogurt, almond milk, maple syrup, and ground cardamom.
2. Blend until it is smooth and creamy.
3. Add ice cubes if a colder consistency is desired and blend again.
4. Pour into glasses and serve immediately.

Serving Suggestions:

- Garnish with a sprinkle of ground cardamom.
- Enjoy as a refreshing beverage or pair with a light snack.

The Cabbage Patch

- **Preparation Time:** 15 minutes
- **Serves:** 2

Ingredients:

- 2 cups green cabbage, finely shredded

- 1 green apple, cored & sliced
- 1 tablespoon fresh lemon juice
- 1 tablespoon honey
- 2 cups cold water
- Ice cubes
- Fresh mint leaves for garnish

Nutritional Information: Calories: 50 | Protein: 1g | Fat: 0g | Carbohydrates: 13g | Fiber: 3g

Instructions:

1. In a large bowl, combine finely shredded green cabbage and thinly sliced green apple.
2. In a separate bowl, mix fresh lemon juice and honey.
3. Pour the lemon-honey mixture over the cabbage and apple, tossing to coat evenly.
4. Divide the cabbage and apple mixture into two glasses.
5. Add cold water to each glass and stir well.
6. Add ice cubes and garnish with fresh mint leaves.

Serving Suggestions:

- Adjust honey and lemon juice to taste.

- Serve as a refreshing alternative to sugary drinks.

CHAPTER 3

30 days Meal Plan for Acid Reflux Diet

Please note that the provided meal plan is a sample and should not be interpreted as a recommendation to consume all the listed recipes in a single day.

This meal plan aims to offer inspiration and guidance for healthy meal preparation. Feel free to customize this plan to suit your preferences and dietary requirements.

Day 1:

- **Breakfast:** Tropical Oatmeal
- **Lunch:** Tortilla wrap with baked omelet
- **Dinner:** Vegetarian Sausage with Braised Cabbage
- **Dessert/Snack:** Coconut & Cacao Loaf

Day 2:

- **Breakfast:** Whole Grain English Muffin
- **Lunch:** Couscous with cod fish
- **Dinner:** Polenta with Sesame Seeds
- **Dessert/Snack:** Paleo Vanilla Sponge Cake

Day 3:

- **Breakfast:** Fabulous French Toast
- **Lunch:** Lunch burger
- **Dinner:** Apricot Glazed Chicken
- **Dessert/Snack:** Cherry & Almond Clafoutis

Day 4:

- **Breakfast:** Easy Vegan Quinoa Breakfast
- **Lunch:** Sweet white rice pudding
- **Dinner:** Banh Mi Bowls with Sticky Tofu
- **Dessert/Snack:** Blueberry Banana Smoothie

Day 5:

- **Breakfast:** Skillet Harvest Pumpkin Hash
- **Lunch:** Bacon, pear, and fig grilled cheese
- **Dinner:** Green Pizza with Pesto, Feta, Artichokes, and Broccoli
- **Dessert/Snack:** Bagel and Lox

Day 6:

- **Breakfast:** Grain-Free Cinnamon Apple Granola
- **Lunch:** White Bean & Avocado Toast
- **Dinner:** Seared Scallops with Acorn Squash Mash
- **Dessert/Snack:** Coconut & Cacao Loaf

Day 7:

- **Breakfast:** Maple Sage Breakfast Patties
- **Lunch:** Rainbow Veggie Wraps
- **Dinner:** Mediterranean Farro Salad with Arugula and Chickpeas
- **Dessert/Snack:** Paleo Vanilla Sponge Cake

Day 8:

- **Breakfast:** Tropical Oatmeal
- **Lunch:** Tortilla wrap with baked omelet
- **Dinner:** Vegetarian Sausage with Braised Cabbage
- **Dessert/Snack:** Coconut & Cacao Loaf

Day 9:

- **Breakfast:** Whole Grain English Muffin
- **Lunch:** Couscous with cod fish
- **Dinner:** Polenta with Sesame Seeds
- **Dessert/Snack:** Paleo Vanilla Sponge Cake

Day 10:

- **Breakfast:** Fabulous French Toast
- **Lunch:** Lunch burger
- **Dinner:** Apricot Glazed Chicken
- **Dessert/Snack:** Cherry & Almond Clafoutis

Day 11:

- **Breakfast:** Easy Vegan Quinoa Breakfast
- **Lunch:** Sweet white rice pudding
- **Dinner:** Banh Mi Bowls with Sticky Tofu
- **Dessert/Snack:** Blueberry Banana Smoothie

Day 12:

- **Breakfast:** Skillet Harvest Pumpkin Hash
- **Lunch:** Bacon, pear, and fig grilled cheese

- **Dinner:** Green Pizza with Pesto, Feta, Artichokes, and Broccoli
- **Dessert/Snack:** Bagel and Lox

Day 13:

- **Breakfast:** Grain-Free Cinnamon Apple Granola
- **Lunch:** White Bean & Avocado Toast
- **Dinner:** Seared Scallops with Acorn Squash Mash
- **Dessert/Snack:** Coconut & Cacao Loaf

Day 14:

- **Breakfast:** Maple Sage Breakfast Patties
- **Lunch:** Rainbow Veggie Wraps
- **Dinner:** Mediterranean Farro Salad with Arugula and Chickpeas
- **Dessert/Snack:** Paleo Vanilla Sponge Cake

Day 15:

- **Breakfast:** Tropical Oatmeal
- **Lunch:** Tortilla wrap with baked omelet
- **Dinner:** Vegetarian Sausage with Braised Cabbage
- **Dessert/Snack:** Coconut & Cacao Loaf

Day 16:

- **Breakfast:** Whole Grain English Muffin
- **Lunch:** Couscous with cod fish
- **Dinner:** Polenta with Sesame Seeds
- **Dessert/Snack:** Paleo Vanilla Sponge Cake

Day 17:

- **Breakfast:** Fabulous French Toast
- **Lunch:** Lunch burger
- **Dinner:** Apricot Glazed Chicken
- **Dessert/Snack:** Cherry & Almond Clafoutis

Day 18:

- **Breakfast:** Easy Vegan Quinoa Breakfast
- **Lunch:** Sweet white rice pudding
- **Dinner:** Banh Mi Bowls with Sticky Tofu
- **Dessert/Snack:** Blueberry Banana Smoothie

Day 19:

- **Breakfast:** Skillet Harvest Pumpkin Hash
- **Lunch:** Bacon, pear, and fig grilled cheese

- **Dinner:** Green Pizza with Pesto, Feta, Artichokes, and Broccoli
- **Dessert/Snack:** Bagel and Lox

Day 20:

- **Breakfast:** Grain-Free Cinnamon Apple Granola
- **Lunch:** White Bean & Avocado Toast
- **Dinner:** Seared Scallops with Acorn Squash Mash
- **Dessert/Snack:** Coconut & Cacao Loaf

Day 21:

- **Breakfast:** Maple Sage Breakfast Patties
- **Lunch:** Rainbow Veggie Wraps
- **Dinner:** Mediterranean Farro Salad with Arugula and Chickpeas
- **Dessert/Snack:** Paleo Vanilla Sponge Cake

Day 22:

- **Breakfast:** Tropical Oatmeal
- **Lunch:** Tortilla wrap with baked omelet
- **Dinner:** Vegetarian Sausage with Braised Cabbage
- **Dessert/Snack:** Coconut & Cacao Loaf

Day 23:

- **Breakfast:** Whole Grain English Muffin
- **Lunch:** Couscous with cod fish
- **Dinner:** Polenta with Sesame Seeds
- **Dessert/Snack:** Paleo Vanilla Sponge Cake

Day 24:

- **Breakfast:** Fabulous French Toast
- **Lunch:** Lunch burger
- **Dinner:** Apricot Glazed Chicken
- **Dessert/Snack:** Cherry & Almond Clafoutis

Day 25:

- **Breakfast:** Easy Vegan Quinoa Breakfast
- **Lunch:** Sweet white rice pudding
- **Dinner:** Banh Mi Bowls with Sticky Tofu
- **Dessert/Snack:** Blueberry Banana Smoothie

Day 26:

- **Breakfast:** Skillet Harvest Pumpkin Hash
- **Lunch:** Bacon, pear, and fig grilled cheese

- **Dinner:** Green Pizza with Pesto, Feta, Artichokes, and Broccoli
- **Dessert/Snack:** Bagel and Lox

Day 27:

- **Breakfast:** Grain-Free Cinnamon Apple Granola
- **Lunch:** White Bean & Avocado Toast
- **Dinner:** Seared Scallops with Acorn Squash Mash
- **Dessert/Snack:** Coconut & Cacao Loaf

Day 28:

- **Breakfast:** Maple Sage Breakfast Patties
- **Lunch:** Rainbow Veggie Wraps
- **Dinner:** Mediterranean Farro Salad with Arugula and Chickpeas
- **Dessert/Snack:** Paleo Vanilla Sponge Cake

Day 29:

- **Breakfast:** Tropical Oatmeal
- **Lunch:** Tortilla wrap with baked omelet
- **Dinner:** Vegetarian Sausage with Braised Cabbage
- **Dessert/Snack:** Coconut & Cacao Loaf

Day 30:

- **Breakfast:** Whole Grain English Muffin
- **Lunch:** Couscous with cod fish
- **Dinner:** Polenta with Sesame Seeds
- **Dessert/Snack:** Paleo Vanilla Sponge Cake

CHAPTER 4

Conclusion

In concluding this Acid Reflux Cookbook for Beginners, our journey through the intricate yet flavorful realm of acid reflux-friendly meals has been a culinary adventure aimed at enhancing not only our digestive well-being but also our enjoyment of food.

As we close the pages of this cookbook, it's important to reflect on the principles, recipes, and the overall impact they can have on our lives.

The principles of the Acid Reflux Diet have guided us towards a mindful and health-centric approach to eating.

By understanding the importance of choosing the right foods and avoiding triggers, we've empowered ourselves to take control of our digestive health.

These principles serve not only as a guide for managing acid reflux but also as a foundation for a wholesome and balanced lifestyle.

The diverse array of recipes provided in this cookbook showcases that an acid reflux-friendly diet need not be bland or restrictive.

From the comforting breakfast to the savory lunch and the delightful dinner, each recipe has been crafted with care, ensuring that flavor is never compromised.

These recipes are a testament to the fact that managing acid reflux doesn't mean sacrificing the joy of eating.

As we peruse the 30-day meal plan, it becomes evident that variety is not only the spice of life but also a key component in maintaining a sustainable and enjoyable dietary regimen.

The rotation of these carefully curated recipes ensures that monotony is replaced with excitement, making the journey towards digestive health an engaging and flavorsome experience.

In essence, this cookbook is not just a collection of recipes but a tool for transformation. It invites you to embark on a culinary exploration that not only addresses acid reflux concerns but also nurtures a love for wholesome, delicious food.

Let this cookbook be a companion on your journey to improved digestive health and a source of inspiration for crafting meals that nourish both body and soul.

May your kitchen continue to be a space where health and happiness converge, one recipe at a time.